I0096634

This publication is intended to provide educational information for the reader on the covered subjects. It is not intended to take the place of personalized medical counseling, diagnosis, and treatment from a trained healthcare professional.

ISBN 978-1-998455-35-5 (Paperback)
ISBN 978-1-998455-36-2 (eBook)

Printed and bound in USA
Published by Loons Press

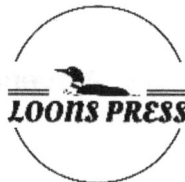

LOONS PRESS

Table Of Contents

How To Heal UTI Naturally

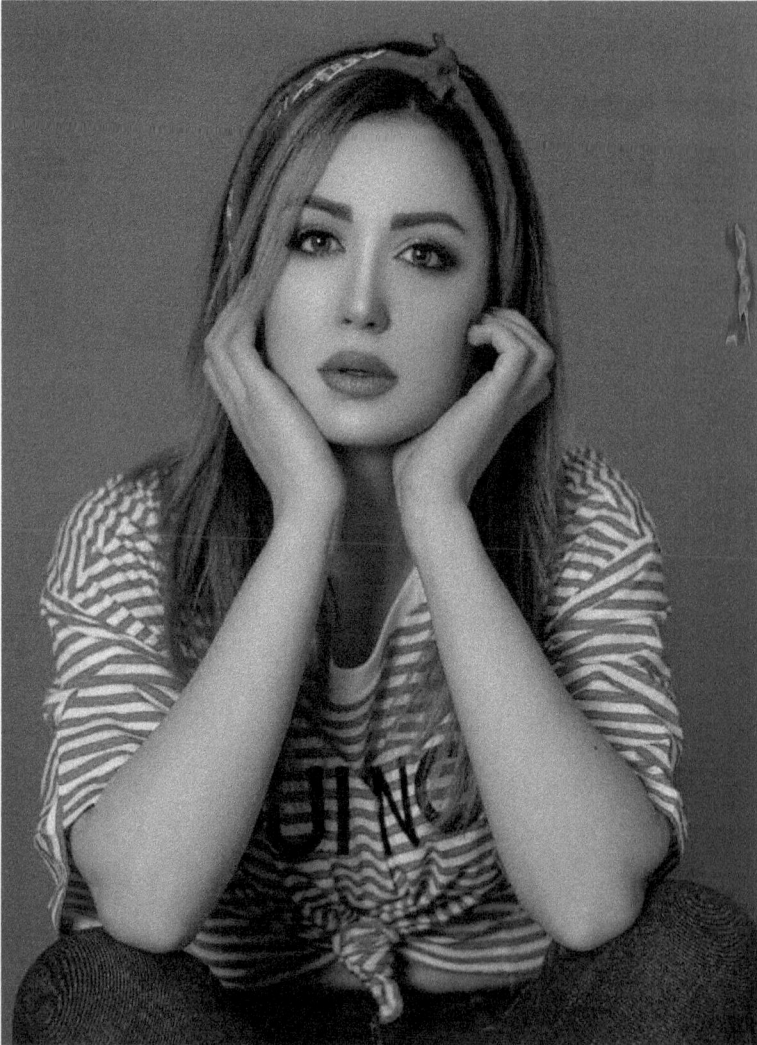

A Comprehensive Guide for Quick Recovery

Chapter 1

Understanding UTI

What is UTI?

Urinary Tract Infections (UTIs) are a common and uncomfortable condition that affects millions of people every year. UTIs occur when bacteria enter the urinary tract and multiply, causing inflammation and infection. Symptoms of UTIs can include a frequent urge to urinate, pain or burning during urination, and cloudy or bloody urine. While UTIs are typically treated with antibiotics, many people are turning to natural remedies for relief.

One of the first steps in healing a UTI naturally is to increase your water intake. Staying hydrated helps to flush out bacteria and toxins from the urinary tract, reducing the risk of infection. Drinking plenty of water also helps to dilute urine, making it less irritating to the bladder and urethra. Aim to drink at least 8-10 glasses of water per day to help prevent and heal UTIs.

Another natural remedy for UTIs is to consume cranberry juice or take cranberry supplements. Cranberries contain compounds that help to prevent bacteria from adhering to the walls of the urinary tract, reducing the risk of infection.

Drinking cranberry juice or taking supplements regularly can help to prevent UTIs from recurring and can also aid in healing existing infections. Be sure to choose unsweetened cranberry juice or supplements to avoid added sugars, which can exacerbate UTI symptoms.

In addition to increasing water intake and consuming cranberry products, there are several other natural remedies that can help to heal UTIs. Probiotics, which are beneficial bacteria that support gut health, can also help to balance the bacteria in the urinary tract and promote healing.

You can find probiotics in supplement form or in foods like yogurt, kefir, and sauerkraut. Herbal remedies like uva ursi, goldenseal, and D-mannose have also been shown to be effective in treating UTIs and promoting urinary tract health.

While natural remedies can be effective in healing UTIs, it is important to consult with a healthcare provider if you suspect you have a UTI. In some cases, UTIs can lead to more serious complications if left untreated, so it is important to seek medical attention if you are experiencing severe symptoms or if your symptoms do not improve with natural remedies.

By taking a holistic approach to healing UTIs, you can not only find relief from uncomfortable symptoms but also support your overall health and well-being.

Causes of UTI

If you are suffering from a urinary tract infection (UTI), it is important to understand the causes of this common and painful condition. UTIs are typically caused by bacteria entering the urinary tract and multiplying, leading to infection.

There are several factors that can increase your risk of developing a UTI, including poor hygiene, sexual activity, and certain medical conditions.

One of the most common causes of UTIs is poor hygiene. Not properly cleaning the genital area can allow bacteria to enter the urinary tract and cause an infection. It is important to always wipe from front to back after using the bathroom to prevent bacteria from entering the urethra.

Additionally, not drinking enough water can also increase your risk of developing a UTI, as dehydration can lead to concentrated urine that allows bacteria to thrive.

Another common cause of UTIs is sexual activity. The friction and movement during intercourse can push bacteria into the urethra, increasing the risk of infection. It is important to urinate before and after sex to help flush out any bacteria that may have entered the urinary tract. Using condoms and practicing good hygiene can also help reduce your risk of developing a UTI after sexual activity.

Certain medical conditions can also increase your risk of developing a UTI. Conditions that affect the immune system, such as diabetes or HIV, can make it harder for your body to fight off infections.

Additionally, conditions that affect the urinary tract, such as kidney stones or an enlarged prostate, can create an environment that is conducive to bacterial growth. It is important to work with your healthcare provider to manage any underlying medical conditions that may be contributing to your UTIs.

In conclusion, understanding the causes of UTIs can help you take steps to prevent them in the future. By practicing good hygiene, staying hydrated, and managing any underlying medical conditions, you can reduce your risk of developing a UTI. Additionally, making lifestyle changes such as urinating before and after sex and using condoms can help protect you from infection. If you are experiencing recurrent UTIs, it is important to speak with your healthcare provider to determine the underlying cause and develop a treatment plan.

Symptoms of UTI

If you are experiencing symptoms of a urinary tract infection (UTI), it is important to recognize them so that you can seek treatment promptly.

UTIs are caused by bacteria entering the urinary tract and can result in uncomfortable and sometimes painful symptoms. Common symptoms of UTIs include a frequent urge to urinate, a burning sensation when urinating, cloudy or strong-smelling urine, and pelvic pain. If you are experiencing any of these symptoms, it is important to consult with a healthcare provider to determine the best course of action for treatment.

In addition to the symptoms mentioned above, some individuals may also experience fever, chills, and fatigue as a result of a UTI. These additional symptoms can be indicative of a more severe infection that may require antibiotics for treatment.

It is important to monitor your symptoms closely and seek medical attention if you are experiencing any of these more severe symptoms. Ignoring symptoms of a UTI can lead to complications and more serious health issues if left untreated.

It is important to note that symptoms of a UTI can vary from person to person and may not always be the same in every case. Some individuals may only experience mild symptoms, while others may have more severe symptoms that require immediate medical attention. It is important to listen to your body and seek help if you are experiencing any unusual or persistent symptoms that are concerning to you.

In some cases, individuals may also experience blood in their urine, which can be a sign of a more serious infection or underlying health condition. If you notice blood in your urine or are experiencing any other concerning symptoms, it is important to seek medical attention right away. Your healthcare provider can perform tests to determine the cause of your symptoms and provide appropriate treatment to help you heal and feel better.

Overall, recognizing the symptoms of a UTI is the first step in addressing the infection and seeking treatment. By being aware of the common symptoms associated with UTIs, you can take proactive steps to heal naturally and prevent the infection from worsening.

Remember to consult with a healthcare provider if you are experiencing any concerning symptoms or have questions about your treatment options. Healing UTIs naturally is possible with the right knowledge and support.

Risk factors for UTI

In order to effectively heal UTI naturally, it is important to understand the various risk factors that can contribute to the development of this common and often painful condition. By identifying and addressing these risk factors, individuals can take proactive steps to prevent UTI and promote overall urinary health.

One of the most common risk factors for UTI is poor hygiene practices. Failing to properly clean the genital area, wiping from back to front after using the bathroom, and not changing out of wet clothing promptly can all increase the likelihood of bacterial growth and infection in the urinary tract. By practicing good hygiene habits, individuals can reduce their risk of developing UTI.

Another significant risk factor for UTI is dehydration. When the body is not properly hydrated, urine becomes more concentrated and bacteria are more likely to thrive in the urinary tract. By drinking plenty of water throughout the day, individuals can help flush out bacteria and prevent the development of UTI.

Certain medical conditions, such as diabetes and kidney stones, can also increase the risk of UTI. Individuals with these conditions should work closely with their healthcare provider to manage their condition and reduce their risk of developing UTI.

Additionally, individuals with a weakened immune system, such as those undergoing chemotherapy or living with HIV/AIDS, are more susceptible to UTI and should take extra precautions to protect their urinary health.

Finally, lifestyle factors such as smoking, stress, and poor diet can also contribute to the development of UTI. By quitting smoking, managing stress levels, and eating a balanced diet rich in fruits, vegetables, and whole grains, individuals can support their overall health and reduce their risk of UTI. By addressing these risk factors and adopting healthy habits, individuals can take proactive steps to heal UTI naturally and prevent future infections.

How To Heal UTI Naturally

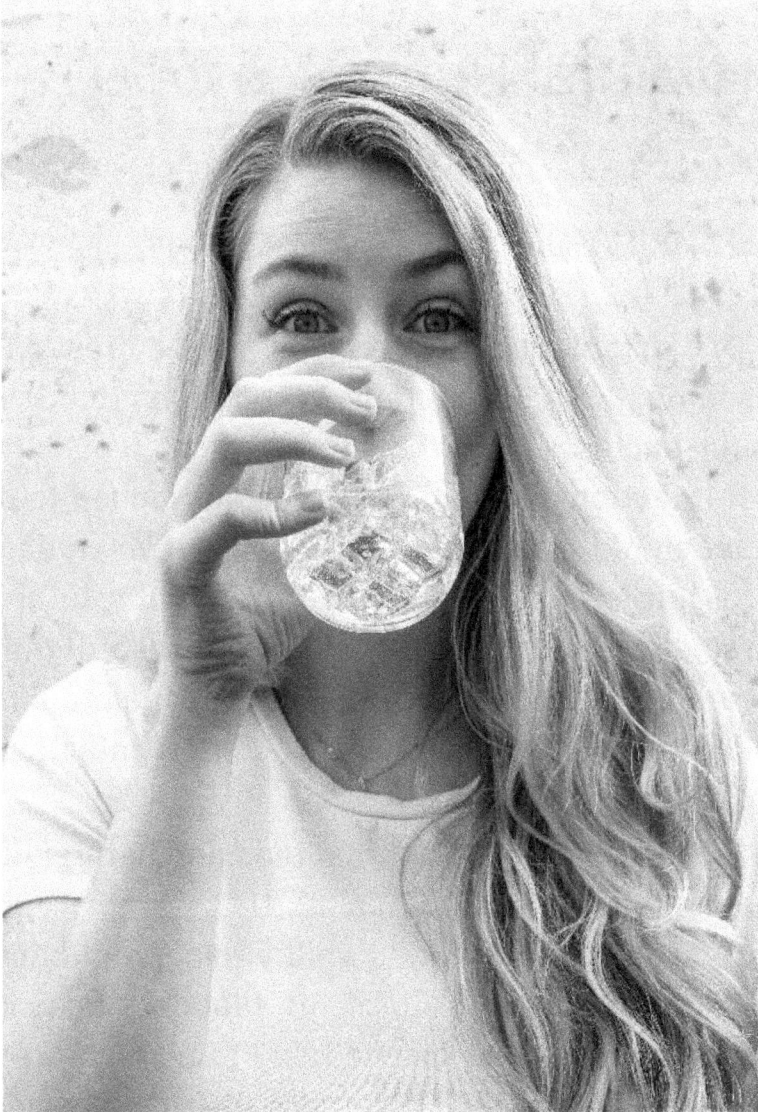

A Comprehensive Guide for Quick Recovery

Chapter 2

Natural Remedies for UTI

Drinking plenty of water

Drinking plenty of water is one of the most crucial steps in healing UTI naturally. Water helps to flush out harmful bacteria from the urinary tract, reducing the risk of infection spreading. It is recommended to drink at least eight glasses of water a day, but when dealing with UTI, it is best to increase that amount to ensure the bacteria are continuously being flushed out of the system. Staying hydrated is key to maintaining a healthy urinary tract and preventing future infections.

In addition to water, herbal teas and natural juices can also be beneficial in healing UTI. Cranberry juice, in particular, is known for its ability to prevent bacteria from sticking to the walls of the bladder and urinary tract, making it easier for the body to eliminate them. Herbal teas like dandelion root and green tea have also been shown to have anti-inflammatory and antibacterial properties that can help in treating UTI naturally.

It is important to avoid drinks that can irritate the bladder and worsen UTI symptoms. This includes alcohol, caffeine, and sugary beverages, as they can all contribute to inflammation and increase the risk of infection. Stick to hydrating, natural drinks like water and herbal teas to support the body's healing process and alleviate discomfort.

For those who struggle to drink enough water throughout the day, setting reminders or carrying a water bottle with you can help you stay on track. Making a conscious effort to prioritize hydration is essential in treating and preventing UTI naturally.

By staying well-hydrated, you are supporting your body's ability to fight off infection and promote overall urinary tract health.

In conclusion, drinking plenty of water is a simple yet effective way to support your body in healing UTI naturally. By staying hydrated and incorporating herbal teas and natural juices into your diet, you can help flush out harmful bacteria and reduce inflammation in the urinary tract.

Remember to avoid irritants like alcohol, caffeine, and sugary drinks, and prioritize hydrating beverages to promote optimal urinary tract health. With a commitment to staying hydrated, you can take control of your UTI symptoms and work towards quick relief and long-term prevention.

Urinate when you need to

Urinary tract infections (UTIs) can be incredibly uncomfortable and disruptive to daily life. One key piece of advice for those suffering from UTIs is to listen to your body and urinate when you need to. Holding in your urine can exacerbate UTI symptoms and prolong the healing process. When you feel the urge to urinate, it is important to do so promptly to help flush out bacteria from your urinary tract.

Many people with UTIs may try to hold their urine for extended periods of time, either due to busy schedules or discomfort while urinating. However, this can actually make UTI symptoms worse. When you hold your urine, bacteria have more time to multiply in your bladder and urinary tract, leading to increased pain and discomfort.

By urinating when you need to, you can help prevent the spread of bacteria and alleviate some of the symptoms associated with UTIs.

In addition to urinating when you feel the urge, it is also important to drink plenty of water throughout the day. Staying hydrated can help to dilute your urine and flush out bacteria more effectively. Aim to drink at least eight glasses of water a day, and be sure to avoid beverages that can irritate the bladder, such as caffeine and alcohol. By staying hydrated and urinating regularly, you can support your body's natural healing process and promote quick relief from UTI symptoms.

If you are having trouble urinating or experiencing pain while doing so, it is important to seek medical attention. Your healthcare provider may recommend medications or other treatments to help alleviate your symptoms and promote healing. In some cases, holding urine may be a sign of a more serious issue, such as a urinary obstruction, that requires immediate attention. By listening to your body and seeking medical advice when needed, you can effectively manage your UTI and promote a speedy recovery.

Overall, urinating when you need to is a simple yet crucial step in healing UTIs naturally. By paying attention to your body's signals and staying hydrated, you can help to flush out bacteria and alleviate discomfort associated with UTIs. Remember to prioritize your health and well-being by taking care of your urinary tract and seeking medical attention when necessary. With the right approach, you can find quick relief and get back to feeling like yourself again.

Avoid irritating foods and drinks

When dealing with a UTI, it is important to be mindful of the foods and drinks you consume as some can exacerbate symptoms and irritate the bladder. Avoiding certain foods and drinks can help alleviate discomfort and promote healing.

One of the main culprits to avoid is caffeine, found in coffee, tea, and soda. Caffeine is a diuretic that can irritate the bladder and worsen UTI symptoms. It is best to opt for caffeine-free alternatives such as herbal tea or water.

Another common irritant for those with UTIs is alcohol. Alcohol can irritate the bladder and increase the frequency of urination, which can be uncomfortable for those already dealing with UTI symptoms. It is best to avoid alcohol while recovering from a UTI and opt for hydrating beverages such as water or herbal teas instead. Alcohol can also dehydrate the body, making it harder for the immune system to fight off the infection.

Spicy foods are another irritant to avoid when dealing with a UTI. Spicy foods can irritate the bladder and exacerbate symptoms such as burning during urination. It is best to steer clear of spicy foods while recovering from a UTI and opt for milder options instead. This includes avoiding hot peppers, chili powder, and other spicy seasonings that can trigger discomfort.

In addition to caffeine, alcohol, and spicy foods, it is also important to avoid acidic foods and drinks such as citrus fruits and juices. Acidic foods can further irritate the bladder and worsen UTI symptoms.

It is best to avoid citrus fruits such as oranges, lemons, and grapefruits, as well as their juices, until the infection has cleared. Opt for alkaline foods such as bananas, leafy greens, and whole grains instead to help soothe the bladder and promote healing.

In conclusion, being mindful of the foods and drinks you consume is essential when dealing with a UTI. Avoiding irritants such as caffeine, alcohol, spicy foods, and acidic foods can help alleviate discomfort and promote healing. Opt for hydrating beverages such as water and herbal tea, and choose alkaline foods to soothe the bladder and support the body's natural healing process. By avoiding irritating foods and drinks, you can help speed up recovery and prevent future UTIs.

Use probiotics to promote good bacteria

If you are someone who suffers from UTIs frequently, you may be familiar with the discomfort and pain that comes with these infections.

UTIs are typically caused by bacteria entering the urinary tract and multiplying, leading to symptoms such as burning during urination, frequent urges to urinate, and cloudy or strong-smelling urine. While antibiotics are often prescribed to treat UTIs, they can also disrupt the balance of good bacteria in the body, leading to further complications. One natural way to promote good bacteria and support your urinary tract health is by using probiotics.

Probiotics are live bacteria and yeasts that are good for your health, especially your digestive system. They are often referred to as "good" or "friendly" bacteria because they help maintain the natural balance of organisms in the intestines. When it comes to UTIs, probiotics can help by restoring the balance of bacteria in the urinary tract, which can help prevent the overgrowth of harmful bacteria that can lead to infections.

One of the most common probiotics used to support urinary tract health is Lactobacillus. This strain of bacteria is naturally found in the body and is known for its ability to promote good bacteria in the gut and urinary tract.

By taking a probiotic supplement containing Lactobacillus, you can help replenish the good bacteria in your body and support your immune system in fighting off harmful bacteria that can cause UTIs.

In addition to taking probiotic supplements, you can also incorporate probiotic-rich foods into your diet to promote good bacteria in your body. Foods such as yogurt, kefir, sauerkraut, and kimchi are all rich sources of probiotics that can help support your urinary tract health. By adding these foods to your diet regularly, you can help maintain a healthy balance of bacteria in your body and reduce your risk of developing UTIs.

Overall, using probiotics to promote good bacteria is a natural and effective way to support your urinary tract health and reduce your risk of developing UTIs. By incorporating probiotic supplements and probiotic-rich foods into your daily routine, you can help restore the balance of bacteria in your body and maintain a healthy urinary tract. Remember to speak with your healthcare provider before starting any new supplements to ensure they are safe and appropriate for your individual needs.

Herbal remedies for UTI

If you're suffering from a UTI, you may be looking for natural remedies to help alleviate your symptoms. Herbal remedies can be a great option for treating UTIs, as they can help to reduce inflammation, fight off bacteria, and promote overall urinary tract health. In this subchapter, we will explore some of the most effective herbal remedies for UTI that you can incorporate into your daily routine.

One of the most popular herbal remedies for UTI is cranberry extract. Cranberries contain compounds that can help to prevent bacteria from sticking to the walls of the urinary tract, reducing the likelihood of infection. You can take cranberry extract in supplement form or drink unsweetened cranberry juice to help promote urinary tract health.

Another powerful herbal remedy for UTI is D-mannose. D-mannose is a type of sugar that can help to prevent bacteria from adhering to the walls of the urinary tract, making it easier for your body to flush out harmful bacteria.

You can find D-mannose supplements at most health food stores, or you can incorporate D-mannose-rich foods like cranberries, apples, and peaches into your diet.

Uva ursi is another herbal remedy that has been used for centuries to treat UTIs. Uva ursi contains compounds that have antibacterial properties, making it an effective treatment for urinary tract infections. You can take uva ursi supplements or drink uva ursi tea to help alleviate your UTI symptoms.

Goldenseal is another herbal remedy that can help to treat UTIs. Goldenseal contains berberine, a compound that has been shown to have antibacterial properties. You can take goldenseal supplements or drink goldenseal tea to help promote urinary tract health and fight off infections.

Incorporating these herbal remedies into your daily routine can help to alleviate your UTI symptoms and promote overall urinary tract health. However, it's important to consult with a healthcare professional before starting any new herbal remedies, especially if you are pregnant, breastfeeding, or taking medications.

By taking a holistic approach to treating your UTI, you can help to alleviate your symptoms and prevent future infections.

How To Heal UTI Naturally

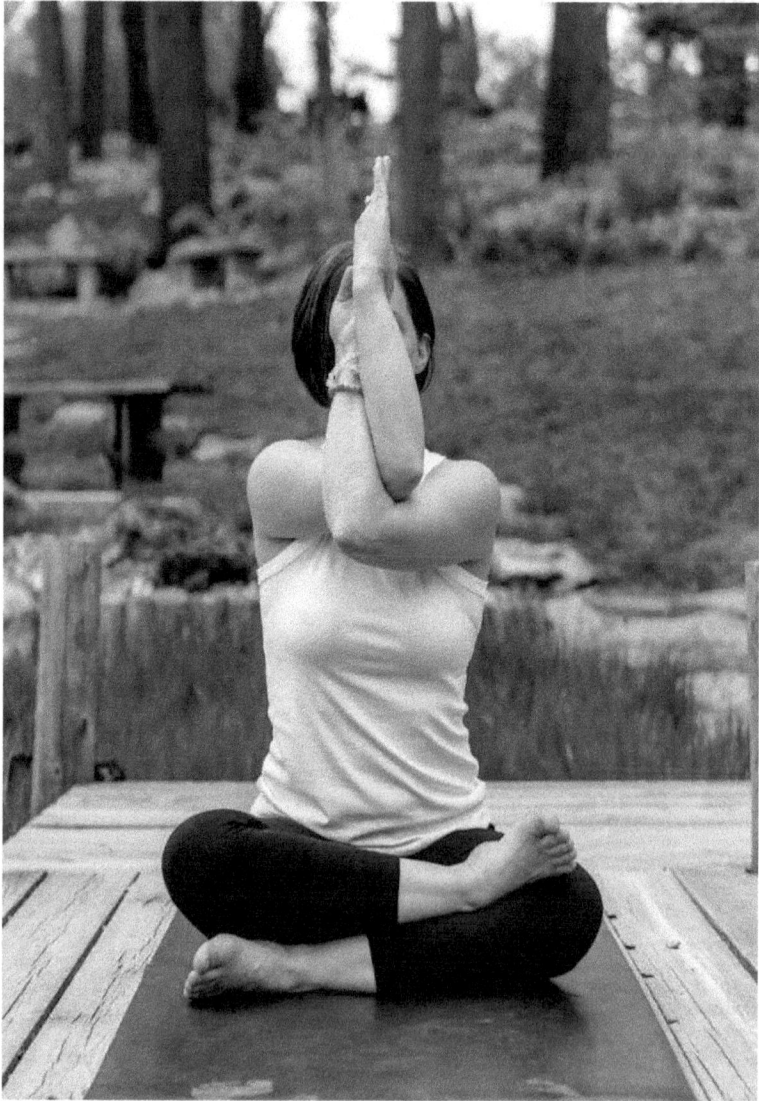

Chapter 3

Lifestyle Changes for UTI Prevention

Wearing cotton underwear

Wearing cotton underwear is an essential step in healing UTI naturally. Cotton is a breathable fabric that allows air to circulate around the genital area, reducing moisture and preventing the growth of bacteria. Synthetic materials, on the other hand, trap moisture and create a warm, damp environment that is perfect for bacteria to thrive. By choosing cotton underwear, you can help keep your genital area dry and reduce the risk of UTI recurrence.

It is important to wear loose-fitting cotton underwear to allow for proper air circulation. Tight-fitting underwear can constrict the genitals and trap moisture, creating an ideal environment for bacteria to multiply. Opt for underwear that is not only made of cotton but also fits comfortably and does not rub or irritate the skin. By choosing the right underwear, you can promote healing and prevent future UTIs.

In addition to wearing cotton underwear, it is also important to practice good hygiene habits. Make sure to change your underwear daily and wash them in hot water to kill any bacteria that may be present. Avoid using scented laundry detergents or fabric softeners, as these can irritate the skin and disrupt the natural balance of bacteria in the genital area.

By maintaining good hygiene practices, you can help support your body's natural ability to fight off UTIs.

For those prone to UTIs, it may be beneficial to wear cotton underwear during the night as well. This can help prevent moisture build-up while you sleep and reduce the risk of developing a UTI.

Additionally, avoid wearing tight clothing or synthetic materials to bed, as these can trap heat and moisture, creating an environment that is conducive to bacterial growth. By making small changes to your bedtime routine, you can support your body's healing process and reduce the likelihood of experiencing a UTI.

Overall, wearing cotton underwear is a simple yet effective way to support your body's natural healing process and prevent UTIs. By choosing breathable, comfortable underwear made of cotton and practicing good hygiene habits, you can reduce the risk of recurrent infections and promote overall urinary tract health. Take care of your body by making small changes to your daily routine, and enjoy the benefits of natural healing and relief from UTIs.

Proper hygiene practices

Proper hygiene practices are crucial for preventing and managing UTIs. One of the most important things you can do is to always wipe from front to back after using the restroom. This helps prevent bacteria from the anus from entering the urethra and causing an infection.

Additionally, it is important to keep the genital area clean and dry, as moist environments can promote bacterial growth.

Another important aspect of proper hygiene is staying hydrated. Drinking plenty of water helps flush out bacteria from the urinary tract and can help prevent UTIs from occurring. Aim to drink at least 8-10 glasses of water per day to keep your urinary system healthy and functioning properly.

It is also important to practice good bathroom habits, such as emptying your bladder completely each time you urinate. Holding in urine for long periods of time can increase the risk of UTIs, as bacteria can multiply in stagnant urine. Make sure to urinate as soon as you feel the urge to go, and don't rush the process to ensure you are fully emptying your bladder.

In addition to proper hygiene practices, wearing loose-fitting, breathable clothing can also help prevent UTIs. Tight clothing can create a warm, moist environment that is ideal for bacterial growth. Opt for cotton underwear and avoid wearing tight pants or leggings for extended periods of time to keep your genital area dry and free from bacteria.

Overall, practicing good hygiene habits is essential for preventing and managing UTIs. By following these simple tips, you can reduce your risk of developing a urinary tract infection and promote overall urinary health. Remember to always consult with a healthcare professional if you are experiencing symptoms of a UTI or have any concerns about your urinary health.

Avoiding douching

In order to effectively heal UTI naturally, it is important to understand the potential dangers of douching. Douching is a common practice among many people with UTIs, but it can actually do more harm than good. Douching involves using a solution to clean out the vagina, but this can disrupt the natural balance of bacteria in the urinary tract, making it easier for infections to occur.

One of the main reasons to avoid douching when dealing with a UTI is that it can actually worsen the symptoms of the infection. The harsh chemicals in many douching solutions can irritate the delicate tissues of the urinary tract, leading to increased pain, burning, and discomfort.

Additionally, douching can also push bacteria further up into the urinary tract, making the infection spread and become more severe.

Another important reason to avoid douching is that it can disrupt the natural balance of bacteria in the urinary tract. The vagina and urinary tract are home to a delicate ecosystem of bacteria that help to keep infections at bay. When this balance is disrupted by douching, it can make it easier for harmful bacteria to multiply and cause UTIs. Instead of douching, it is better to focus on natural remedies and treatments that support the body's own ability to fight off infections.

If you are dealing with a UTI, it is important to avoid douching and instead focus on natural ways to heal your body. Drinking plenty of water, eating a healthy diet rich in fruits and vegetables, and getting plenty of rest can all help to support your body's natural healing process. Additionally, there are many natural remedies that can help to alleviate the symptoms of a UTI and promote healing, such as cranberry juice, probiotics, and herbal supplements.

By avoiding douching and focusing on natural remedies and treatments, you can effectively heal your UTI and prevent future infections. Remember to listen to your body, stay hydrated, and give yourself the rest and care you need to recover fully. With a holistic approach to healing, you can successfully overcome UTIs and enjoy better urinary health in the long run.

Urinate after intercourse

Urinary tract infections (UTIs) are a common and painful condition that can affect anyone, but they are more common in women. One important step in preventing UTIs is to urinate after intercourse. During sex, bacteria can be pushed into the urethra, increasing the risk of infection. By emptying your bladder after sex, you can help flush out any bacteria that may have entered the urinary tract.

It is crucial to urinate within 15 minutes of intercourse to effectively reduce the risk of developing a UTI. Holding in your urine for an extended period after sex can allow bacteria to multiply and increase the chances of an infection.

Additionally, drinking plenty of water before and after intercourse can help dilute the urine and flush out any bacteria that may be present.

In addition to urinating after intercourse, there are other natural methods you can use to help prevent and treat UTIs. Drinking cranberry juice or taking cranberry supplements can help prevent bacteria from sticking to the walls of the bladder, reducing the risk of infection. Probiotics can also help maintain a healthy balance of good bacteria in the gut and urinary tract, preventing the overgrowth of harmful bacteria that can lead to UTIs.

It is essential to practice good hygiene habits to prevent UTIs, such as wiping from front to back after using the bathroom and wearing cotton underwear to allow the area to breathe.

Avoiding irritating products like douches, scented soaps, and tight clothing can also help reduce the risk of UTIs. By following these natural methods and lifestyle changes, you can help prevent UTIs and promote overall urinary tract health.

If you are experiencing symptoms of a UTI, such as a frequent urge to urinate, burning sensation when urinating, or cloudy urine, it is essential to see a healthcare professional for proper diagnosis and treatment. In some cases, antibiotics may be necessary to clear the infection. However, by incorporating these natural methods into your routine, you can reduce the frequency of UTIs and promote overall urinary tract health.

Managing stress levels

Managing stress levels is crucial for individuals dealing with UTI. Stress can weaken the immune system, making it harder for the body to fight off infections like UTI. Therefore, it is important to find ways to reduce stress in order to promote healing and prevent future infections.

One effective way to manage stress levels is through relaxation techniques such as deep breathing, meditation, or yoga. These practices can help calm the mind and body, allowing for better stress management and well-being. Taking time each day to practice these techniques can have a significant impact on reducing stress and improving overall health.

In addition to relaxation techniques, regular exercise can also help manage stress levels. Exercise releases endorphins, which are chemicals in the brain that act as natural painkillers and mood elevators. By incorporating regular physical activity into your routine, you can reduce stress and improve your overall mental and physical health.

Another important aspect of managing stress levels is maintaining a healthy lifestyle. This includes eating a balanced diet, getting enough sleep, and staying hydrated. By taking care of your body through proper nutrition and self-care, you can better equip yourself to handle stress and prevent UTI infections.

Overall, managing stress levels is a key component of healing UTI naturally. By incorporating relaxation techniques, exercise, and healthy lifestyle habits into your daily routine, you can reduce stress, boost your immune system, and promote healing from UTI. Remember to prioritize self-care and stress management in order to support your overall health and well-being.

How To Heal UTI Naturally

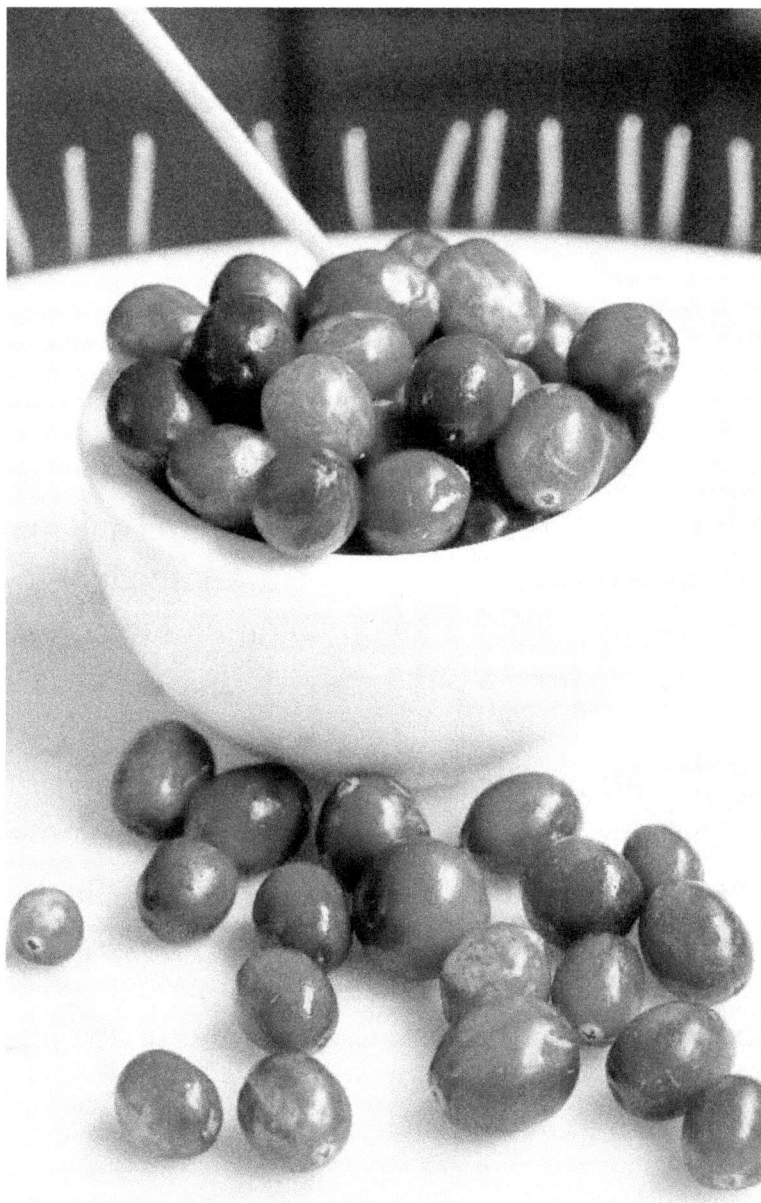

Chapter 4

Dietary Recommendations for UTI

Foods to avoid

When dealing with a urinary tract infection (UTI), it's important to be mindful of the foods you consume. Some foods can aggravate your symptoms and make it harder for your body to fight off the infection. In this chapter, we will discuss some common foods to avoid when suffering from a UTI.

First and foremost, it's crucial to stay away from foods that are high in sugar. Sugar can promote the growth of bacteria in your urinary tract, making it more difficult for your body to fight off the infection. This includes sugary drinks, desserts, and processed foods that contain added sugars. Opt for natural sweeteners like honey or stevia instead.

Another food group to avoid when dealing with a UTI is dairy products. Dairy can be difficult for some people to digest, leading to inflammation in the body. This can exacerbate UTI symptoms and prolong the healing process. Try switching to non-dairy alternatives like almond milk or coconut yogurt to see if it helps alleviate your symptoms.

Spicy foods can also be problematic for individuals with UTIs. Spices like chili peppers and hot sauces can irritate the bladder and urethra, causing discomfort and worsening symptoms. If you enjoy spicy foods, try to consume them in moderation or opt for milder alternatives to prevent aggravating your UTI.

Alcohol is another culprit that can worsen UTI symptoms. Alcohol is dehydrating and can irritate the bladder, making it harder for your body to flush out bacteria. It's best to avoid alcohol altogether when dealing with a UTI to give your body the best chance at healing quickly and effectively.

Lastly, it's important to limit your intake of caffeine when suffering from a UTI. Caffeine is a diuretic, meaning it can increase urination and potentially irritate the bladder. This can exacerbate symptoms and make it harder for your body to heal. Opt for caffeine-free alternatives like herbal teas or decaf coffee to help alleviate your symptoms and support the healing process.

Foods to include

In order to effectively treat and prevent UTIs naturally, it is important to incorporate certain foods into your diet. These foods can help to boost your immune system, fight off infection, and promote overall urinary tract health. By including these foods in your daily meals, you can work towards healing your UTI and preventing future infections.

One food that is essential for healing UTIs naturally is cranberries. Cranberries contain compounds that help to prevent bacteria from sticking to the walls of the urinary tract, making it easier for the body to flush out the infection. Drinking cranberry juice or eating fresh cranberries can be a great way to incorporate this superfood into your diet.

Another important food to include in your diet when dealing with a UTI is garlic. Garlic is known for its antimicrobial properties, which can help to fight off the bacteria causing the infection. Adding garlic to your meals or taking garlic supplements can help to speed up the healing process and prevent the infection from spreading.

Probiotic-rich foods, such as yogurt and kefir, can also be beneficial for healing UTIs naturally. Probiotics help to restore the balance of good bacteria in the gut and urinary tract, which can help to prevent the overgrowth of harmful bacteria that can lead to infections. Including these foods in your diet can help to strengthen your immune system and promote overall urinary tract health.

In addition to these specific foods, it is important to stay hydrated when dealing with a UTI. Drinking plenty of water can help to flush out bacteria from the urinary tract and prevent dehydration, which can make symptoms of a UTI worse. Herbal teas, such as dandelion root or green tea, can also be beneficial for promoting urinary tract health and speeding up the healing process.

Overall, incorporating these foods into your diet can help to heal UTIs naturally and prevent future infections. By focusing on whole, nutrient-rich foods that support your immune system and promote urinary tract health, you can work towards quick relief and long-term healing. Remember to consult with a healthcare professional before making any significant changes to your diet or treatment plan.

Importance of vitamin C

Vitamin C is an essential nutrient that plays a crucial role in supporting the immune system and overall health. For people suffering from UTI, increasing their intake of vitamin C can be especially beneficial. Vitamin C is known for its antioxidant properties, which can help to fight off harmful bacteria that cause UTI. By boosting the immune system, vitamin C can help the body to better defend against infections and promote faster healing.

One of the key benefits of vitamin C for UTI sufferers is its ability to acidify the urine. This can help to create an environment in the bladder that is less hospitable to bacteria, making it more difficult for them to thrive and cause infection.

By increasing their intake of vitamin C through foods like citrus fruits, strawberries, and bell peppers, UTI sufferers can help to prevent future infections and promote faster recovery from current ones.

In addition to its role in supporting the immune system and acidifying the urine, vitamin C also has anti-inflammatory properties that can help to reduce the pain and discomfort associated with UTI. By reducing inflammation in the bladder and urinary tract, vitamin C can help to alleviate symptoms like burning urination and frequent urges to urinate. This can make the experience of having UTI more manageable and improve overall quality of life for those suffering from the condition.

It is important for people with UTI to ensure that they are getting an adequate amount of vitamin C in their diet. While vitamin C supplements can be helpful, it is always best to get nutrients from whole foods whenever possible. By incorporating vitamin C-rich foods into their meals and snacks, UTI sufferers can support their immune system, acidify their urine, and reduce inflammation in the bladder and urinary tract.

In conclusion, vitamin C plays a crucial role in supporting the health and well-being of people with UTI. By increasing their intake of vitamin C through foods and supplements, UTI sufferers can help to boost their immune system, acidify their urine, and reduce inflammation in the bladder and urinary tract. This can lead to faster healing, prevention of future infections, and a reduction in symptoms like pain and discomfort. By understanding the importance of vitamin C for UTI, individuals can take proactive steps to improve their overall health and well-being.

Limiting caffeine and alcohol intake

Limiting caffeine and alcohol intake is crucial for those suffering from UTI as both substances can exacerbate symptoms and prolong recovery time. Caffeine is a diuretic that can irritate the bladder and increase the frequency of urination, causing discomfort for those already experiencing UTI symptoms. Alcohol, on the other hand, can dehydrate the body and weaken the immune system, making it harder for the body to fight off the infection. By reducing or eliminating these substances from your diet, you can help your body heal more quickly and effectively.

One way to limit caffeine intake is by switching to decaffeinated versions of your favorite beverages. This can help reduce the irritation to the bladder while still allowing you to enjoy the taste of coffee, tea, or soda.

Additionally, you can explore herbal teas or other caffeine-free alternatives to help satisfy your cravings without worsening your UTI symptoms. It's important to pay attention to how your body responds to different beverages and adjust your intake accordingly.

Similarly, cutting back on alcohol consumption can have a positive impact on your UTI symptoms. Try opting for non-alcoholic beverages or mocktails when socializing with friends or attending events.

By staying hydrated with water or herbal teas instead of alcohol, you can support your body's natural healing process and reduce the risk of recurrent UTIs. Remember that moderation is key, and listening to your body's signals can help you make informed choices about what you consume.

In addition to limiting caffeine and alcohol intake, it's important to focus on staying hydrated with plenty of water throughout the day. Drinking water helps flush out bacteria from the urinary tract and can prevent the formation of kidney stones, which can complicate UTI symptoms. Aim to drink at least eight glasses of water per day, and consider adding lemon or cranberry juice to your water for added benefits. By maintaining proper hydration, you can support your body's ability to heal and prevent future UTIs.

Overall, making conscious choices to limit caffeine and alcohol intake can have a significant impact on your UTI symptoms and overall well-being. By paying attention to how these substances affect your body and adjusting your habits accordingly, you can support your body's natural healing process and reduce the likelihood of recurrent infections. Remember that every person is different, so it's important to listen to your body and work with a healthcare provider to create a personalized plan for managing UTI symptoms. By taking a holistic approach to healing, you can empower yourself to make positive changes that support your health and well-being.

Incorporating cranberry juice

Incorporating cranberry juice into your daily routine can be a powerful way to help heal UTI naturally. Cranberry juice is well-known for its ability to prevent and treat urinary tract infections due to its high levels of antioxidants and compounds that can help prevent bacteria from sticking to the walls of the urinary tract.

When choosing cranberry juice, opt for a pure, unsweetened version to avoid added sugars that can exacerbate UTI symptoms.

One of the most effective ways to incorporate cranberry juice into your routine is to drink a glass of it first thing in the morning and before bed. This can help to flush out bacteria and prevent them from multiplying in your urinary tract.

It is important to drink plenty of water throughout the day as well, as this will help to further flush out bacteria and keep your urinary tract healthy.

You can also mix cranberry juice with water or herbal tea to create a refreshing and healing beverage. Adding a squeeze of lemon or a dash of honey can enhance the taste and provide additional health benefits. Remember to choose a cranberry juice that is 100% pure and free of added sugars, as these can actually worsen UTI symptoms.

In addition to drinking cranberry juice, you can also incorporate it into your diet in other ways. Try adding it to smoothies, yogurt, or oatmeal for a delicious and nutritious boost. You can also use cranberry juice as a base for salad dressings or marinades to add a tangy flavor to your meals while reaping the benefits of its healing properties.

Overall, incorporating cranberry juice into your daily routine is a simple and effective way to help heal UTI naturally. By drinking it regularly and finding creative ways to include it in your diet, you can support your body's natural healing process and prevent future infections. Remember to consult with a healthcare professional if you have any questions or concerns about using cranberry juice as a natural remedy for UTI.

How To Heal UTI Naturally

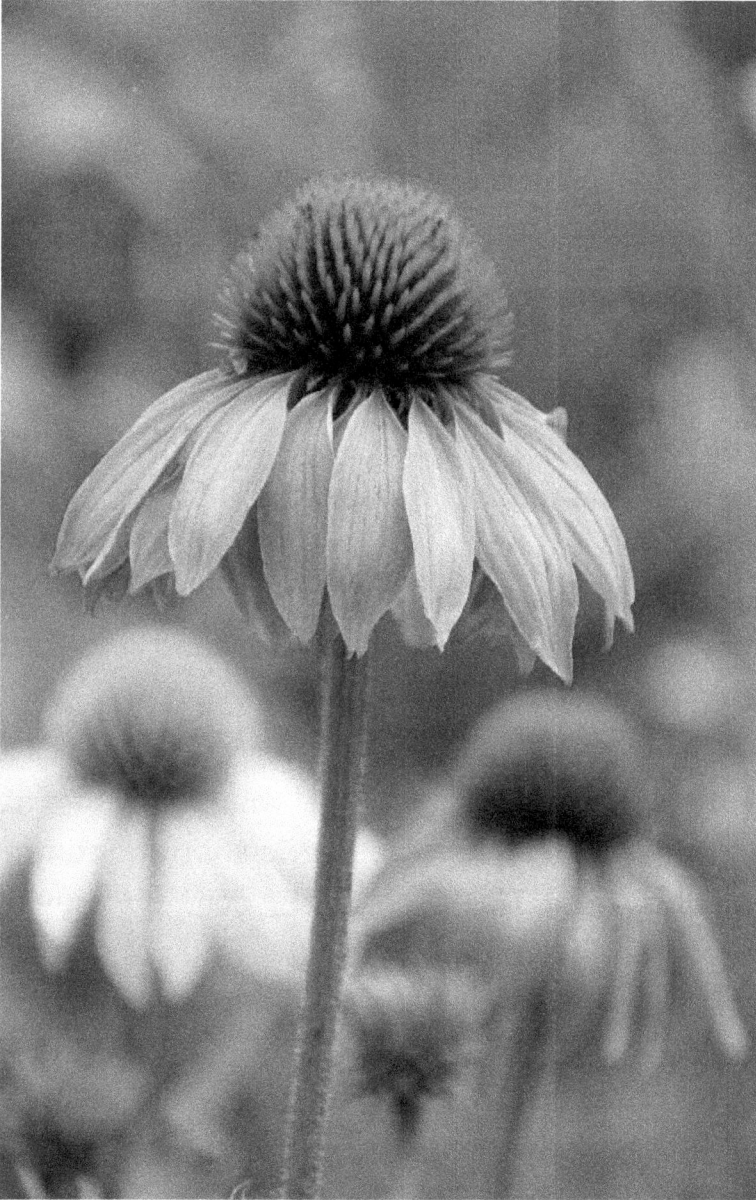

Chapter 5

Supplements for UTI Relief

D-mannose

D-mannose is a natural supplement that has gained popularity in recent years for its ability to help treat urinary tract infections (UTIs) effectively and naturally. It is a type of sugar that is found in fruits like cranberries and acts as a natural antibiotic, helping to prevent bacteria from adhering to the walls of the urinary tract. This makes it a powerful tool in the fight against UTIs, which are often caused by bacteria entering the urinary tract and multiplying.

One of the key benefits of D-mannose is its ability to target specific types of bacteria that are commonly responsible for UTIs, such as E. coli. By preventing these bacteria from sticking to the walls of the urinary tract, D-mannose can help to flush them out of the body more effectively, reducing the severity and frequency of UTI symptoms. This can be particularly useful for people who suffer from recurrent UTIs, as D-mannose can help to break the cycle of infection and provide long-lasting relief.

In addition to its antibacterial properties, D-mannose is also known for its ability to promote a healthy balance of bacteria in the gut and urinary tract. This can help to strengthen the body's natural defenses against infection and support overall urinary tract health.

By incorporating D-mannose into your daily routine, you can help to maintain a healthy urinary tract environment and reduce your risk of developing UTIs in the future.

When using D-mannose to treat a UTI, it is important to follow the recommended dosage instructions and consult with a healthcare provider if you have any underlying health conditions or are taking other medications.

While D-mannose is generally considered safe and well-tolerated, it may not be suitable for everyone. By working with a healthcare provider, you can ensure that you are using D-mannose safely and effectively to help heal your UTI naturally.

Overall, D-mannose is a powerful and natural supplement that can help to provide quick relief from UTI symptoms and support long-term urinary tract health. By incorporating D-mannose into your daily routine, you can take control of your UTI symptoms and reduce your risk of recurrent infections.

With its antibacterial properties and ability to support a healthy urinary tract environment, D-mannose is a valuable tool in the fight against UTIs and can help you to heal naturally and effectively.

Probiotic supplements

Probiotic supplements are a natural and effective way to help heal UTIs. These supplements contain beneficial bacteria that can help restore the balance of good bacteria in the gut and urinary tract, which can be disrupted during a UTI. By taking probiotic supplements, you can help support your body's natural defenses against harmful bacteria and promote overall urinary tract health.

One of the key benefits of probiotic supplements for UTI relief is their ability to help prevent the overgrowth of harmful bacteria in the urinary tract. When the balance of good bacteria in the gut and urinary tract is disrupted, it can create an environment where harmful bacteria can thrive. By taking probiotic supplements, you can help restore this balance and reduce the risk of UTI recurrence.

In addition to helping prevent UTIs, probiotic supplements can also help reduce the severity of symptoms associated with UTIs. Studies have shown that probiotics can help reduce inflammation in the urinary tract and improve the body's ability to fight off infection. By incorporating probiotic supplements into your UTI treatment plan, you may experience faster relief from symptoms such as pain, burning, and frequent urination.

When choosing a probiotic supplement for UTI relief, it is important to look for one that contains strains of bacteria known to be beneficial for urinary tract health, such as Lactobacillus and Bifidobacterium.

It is also important to choose a supplement that is high quality and contains a sufficient number of live bacteria to be effective. Consulting with a healthcare provider or a natural health practitioner can help you determine the best probiotic supplement for your specific needs.

Overall, probiotic supplements can be a valuable addition to a natural UTI treatment plan. By helping to restore the balance of good bacteria in the gut and urinary tract, probiotics can help prevent UTIs, reduce symptoms, and support overall urinary tract health. Incorporating probiotic supplements into your daily routine can be a simple and effective way to promote healing and prevent UTI recurrence.

Vitamin C supplements

Vitamin C supplements play a crucial role in the natural treatment of UTIs. Vitamin C, also known as ascorbic acid, is a powerful antioxidant that helps boost the immune system and fight off infections. When it comes to UTIs, vitamin C can help acidify the urine, making it less hospitable for bacteria to thrive. This can help prevent the spread of infection and promote healing.

One of the most common ways to supplement with vitamin C is through daily capsules or tablets. It is important to choose a high-quality supplement from a reputable source to ensure maximum benefit.

The recommended dosage for UTI prevention and treatment typically ranges from 500-2000mg per day, but it is best to consult with a healthcare provider for personalized recommendations.

In addition to taking vitamin C supplements, incorporating vitamin C-rich foods into your diet can also be beneficial. Citrus fruits like oranges, grapefruits, and lemons are excellent sources of vitamin C. Other fruits and vegetables such as strawberries, kiwi, bell peppers, and broccoli are also great options.

By increasing your intake of these vitamin C-rich foods, you can help support your body's natural defense mechanisms against UTIs.

It is important to note that while vitamin C supplements can be helpful in the treatment of UTIs, they should not be used as a standalone treatment. It is always best to consult with a healthcare provider to determine the best course of action for your individual situation. In some cases, additional treatments such as antibiotics or other natural remedies may be necessary to fully heal a UTI.

Overall, vitamin C supplements can be a valuable tool in the natural treatment of UTIs. By boosting your immune system and acidifying your urine, vitamin C can help prevent and fight off infections. Combined with a healthy diet and other natural remedies, vitamin C supplements can be a key component in your journey to healing UTIs naturally.

Garlic capsules

Garlic capsules have long been touted for their powerful antibacterial properties and ability to boost the immune system, making them a popular choice for those looking to naturally heal UTIs. These capsules contain concentrated amounts of allicin, the active ingredient in garlic that provides its potent antimicrobial effects.

By taking garlic capsules regularly, individuals with UTIs can help to fight off the bacteria causing their infection and promote overall urinary tract health.

One of the key benefits of using garlic capsules to heal UTIs naturally is their ability to target a wide range of bacteria, including the common culprits responsible for urinary tract infections. Studies have shown that garlic has the ability to inhibit the growth of bacteria such as E. coli, which is often the cause of UTIs. By incorporating garlic capsules into their daily routine, individuals can help to prevent the spread of bacteria in the urinary tract and reduce the likelihood of developing recurrent infections.

In addition to their antibacterial properties, garlic capsules also have anti-inflammatory effects that can help to reduce pain and discomfort associated with UTIs. By reducing inflammation in the urinary tract, garlic capsules can provide relief from symptoms such as burning during urination, frequent urination, and pelvic pain. This can make the healing process more comfortable for individuals suffering from UTIs and help them to get back to their daily routines more quickly.

When choosing garlic capsules for UTI relief, it is important to select a high-quality supplement that contains a standardized amount of allicin. This ensures that individuals are receiving a consistent dose of the active ingredient in garlic that provides its therapeutic effects.

It is also recommended to consult with a healthcare provider before starting any new supplement regimen, especially for those with underlying health conditions or who are taking medications that may interact with garlic capsules.

In conclusion, garlic capsules can be a valuable addition to a natural approach to healing UTIs. Their potent antibacterial and anti-inflammatory properties make them a powerful tool for fighting off infections and promoting urinary tract health.

By incorporating garlic capsules into their daily routine, individuals with UTIs can support their body's natural defenses and work towards quick relief and long-term prevention of urinary tract infections.

Echinacea

Echinacea is a popular herbal remedy that has been used for centuries to treat various ailments, including urinary tract infections (UTIs). This powerful herb is known for its immune-boosting properties, making it an excellent choice for those looking to naturally heal their UTI. Echinacea works by stimulating the immune system to help fight off the bacteria causing the infection, while also reducing inflammation and relieving symptoms such as pain and burning during urination.

One of the key benefits of using echinacea to treat a UTI is its ability to target the root cause of the infection, rather than just masking the symptoms. By boosting the body's natural defenses, echinacea can help to prevent future UTIs from occurring, making it a valuable addition to any natural healing regimen.

In addition, echinacea is gentle on the stomach and does not have the same side effects as many prescription medications, making it a safe and effective option for those looking to avoid harsh chemicals and antibiotics.

When using echinacea to treat a UTI, it is important to choose a high-quality supplement that contains a standardized amount of the active ingredient, echinacoside. This ensures that you are getting a potent dose of the herb and will experience maximum benefits.

It is also recommended to consult with a healthcare professional before starting any new herbal remedy, especially if you are pregnant, nursing, or taking other medications.

In addition to taking echinacea supplements, you can also brew echinacea tea to help alleviate symptoms of a UTI. Simply steep a teaspoon of dried echinacea root in a cup of hot water for 10-15 minutes, then strain and drink the tea up to three times a day. This can help to soothe inflammation and reduce pain and discomfort associated with a UTI.

However, it is important to note that echinacea tea should not be used as a substitute for medical treatment, and if symptoms persist or worsen, you should seek medical attention.

Overall, echinacea is a valuable tool in the natural healing arsenal for those suffering from UTIs. By boosting the immune system, reducing inflammation, and relieving symptoms, echinacea can help to provide quick relief and prevent future infections. Whether taken in supplement form or brewed into a soothing tea, echinacea is a safe and effective option for those looking to heal UTIs naturally and avoid the use of antibiotics.

How To Heal UTI Naturally

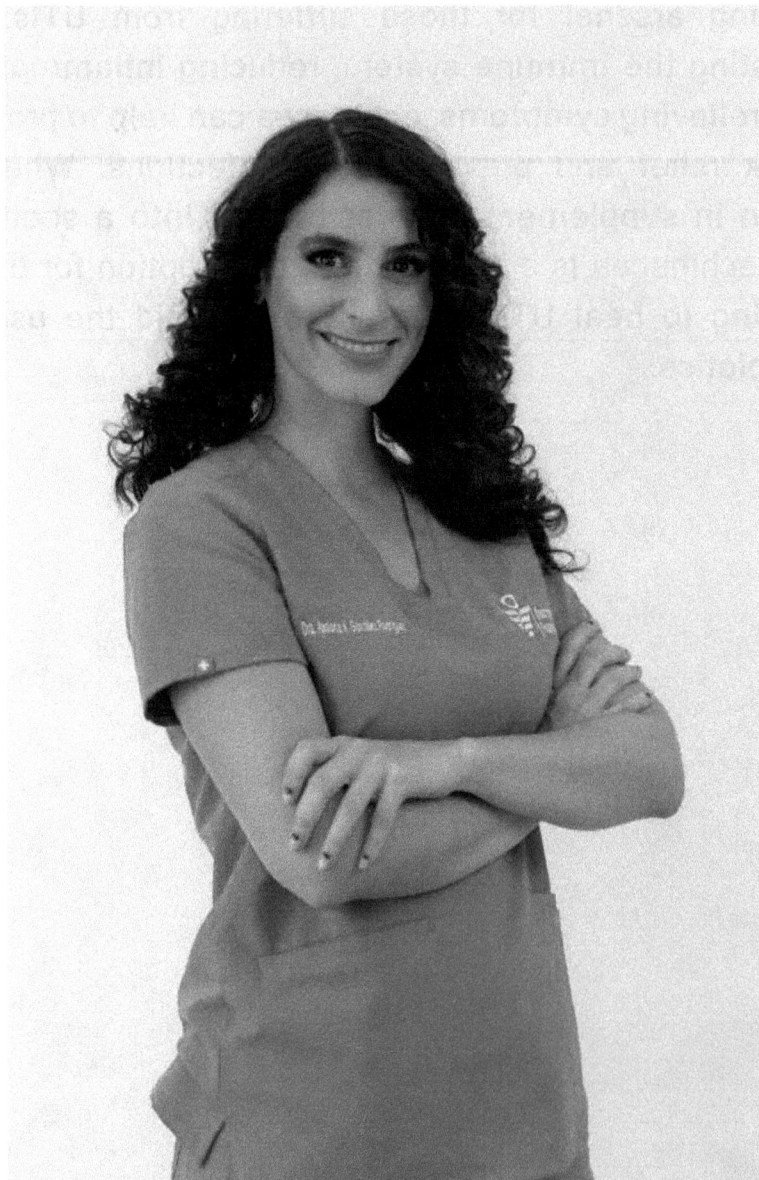

Chapter 6

Seeking Medical Help for UTI

When to see a doctor

When dealing with a urinary tract infection (UTI), it is important to know when it is time to seek medical attention from a doctor. While there are many natural remedies that can help alleviate symptoms and promote healing, sometimes a UTI can become severe and require professional medical intervention. Here are some signs that indicate it may be time to see a doctor for your UTI.

If you are experiencing severe pain or discomfort in your lower abdomen or back, it is important to see a doctor. This could be a sign that the infection has spread to your kidneys, which can lead to more serious complications if left untreated. Additionally, if you have a fever or chills along with your UTI symptoms, this may indicate a more severe infection that requires medical attention.

Another reason to see a doctor for your UTI is if you are not experiencing any relief from your symptoms after trying natural remedies for a few days. While natural remedies can be effective for many people, they may not work for everyone, and it is important to seek medical advice if your symptoms persist.

If you have a history of recurrent UTIs or if you are pregnant, it is also important to see a doctor for your UTI. Recurrent UTIs can be a sign of an underlying issue that may require medical treatment, and UTIs during pregnancy can lead to complications if not properly treated.

Finally, if you are experiencing frequent UTIs or if your symptoms are severe, it is important to see a doctor for a proper diagnosis and treatment plan. UTIs can be uncomfortable and disruptive to your daily life, and seeking medical attention can help you get the relief you need to feel better.

In conclusion, while natural remedies can be effective for treating UTIs, there are times when it is important to see a doctor for your infection. If you are experiencing severe pain, fever, chills, lack of relief from natural remedies, a history of recurrent UTIs, pregnancy, or frequent infections, it is important to seek medical advice to ensure proper treatment and avoid complications.

Remember, your health is important, and it is always better to be safe than sorry when it comes to UTIs.

Diagnostic tests for UTI

In order to properly diagnose a urinary tract infection (UTI), healthcare providers may recommend a variety of diagnostic tests. These tests are crucial in determining the presence of bacteria in the urinary tract and guiding appropriate treatment. Understanding the different diagnostic tests available can help individuals with UTIs navigate their healthcare journey more effectively.

One common diagnostic test for UTIs is a urine culture. This test involves collecting a sample of urine and sending it to a laboratory for analysis. The lab will then grow any bacteria present in the urine to determine the specific type causing the infection. This information is crucial for healthcare providers to prescribe the most effective antibiotic treatment.

Another common diagnostic test for UTIs is a urinalysis. This test involves examining the physical and chemical properties of urine, as well as looking for the presence of white blood cells, red blood cells, and bacteria. A urinalysis can provide valuable information about the severity of the infection and guide treatment decisions.

In some cases, healthcare providers may recommend a urine cytology test. This test involves examining urine under a microscope to look for abnormal cells that may indicate a more serious underlying condition, such as bladder cancer. While UTIs are usually benign, it's important to rule out more serious conditions through diagnostic testing.

Individuals with recurrent UTIs may also undergo imaging tests, such as a CT scan or ultrasound, to evaluate the urinary tract for structural abnormalities that may be contributing to the infections. These tests can help healthcare providers determine the underlying cause of recurrent UTIs and develop a more targeted treatment plan.

Overall, diagnostic tests play a crucial role in the management of UTIs. By understanding the different tests available and their implications, individuals with UTIs can work with their healthcare providers to develop an effective treatment plan and find relief from their symptoms. It's important to communicate openly with healthcare providers about symptoms and concerns to ensure appropriate testing and treatment.

Conventional treatment options

Conventional treatment options for urinary tract infections (UTIs) typically involve the use of antibiotics prescribed by a healthcare provider. While antibiotics can effectively kill the bacteria causing the infection, they may also have negative side effects such as upset stomach, diarrhea, and yeast infections.

It is important to follow your healthcare provider's instructions and complete the full course of antibiotics to fully treat the infection and prevent it from returning.

In addition to antibiotics, healthcare providers may also recommend over-the-counter pain relievers such as ibuprofen or acetaminophen to help alleviate discomfort and reduce fever associated with UTIs. Drinking plenty of water and urinating frequently can also help flush out bacteria from the urinary tract and relieve symptoms. It is important to avoid holding in urine for long periods of time, as this can allow bacteria to multiply and worsen the infection.

For some people who have recurrent UTIs, healthcare providers may recommend a low-dose antibiotic regimen to prevent future infections. This involves taking a small dose of antibiotics daily or after certain activities that may trigger UTIs, such as sexual intercourse.

While this approach can be effective in preventing UTIs, it is important to discuss the potential risks and benefits with your healthcare provider to determine if this is the right option for you.

If conventional treatment options do not provide relief or if you are looking for alternative ways to manage UTIs, there are natural remedies and lifestyle changes that may help. Some people find relief from UTI symptoms by drinking cranberry juice or taking cranberry supplements, as cranberries contain compounds that may prevent bacteria from sticking to the walls of the urinary tract.

Other natural remedies that may help alleviate UTI symptoms include probiotics, garlic, and D-mannose.

It is important to consult with your healthcare provider before trying any natural remedies to ensure they are safe and effective for your specific situation. In some cases, natural remedies may not be enough to fully treat a UTI and conventional treatment options such as antibiotics may still be necessary.

By working with your healthcare provider and exploring different treatment options, you can find the best approach to manage and heal UTIs naturally.

Antibiotic resistance

Antibiotic resistance is a growing concern in the treatment of urinary tract infections (UTIs). As bacteria evolve and develop resistance to commonly prescribed antibiotics, it becomes increasingly difficult to effectively treat these infections. This can lead to recurring UTIs, prolonged symptoms, and even more serious complications. It is crucial for individuals with UTIs to be aware of the risks of antibiotic resistance and explore alternative treatment options.

One of the main causes of antibiotic resistance in UTIs is the overuse and misuse of antibiotics. Many individuals are quick to reach for antibiotics at the first sign of a UTI, without considering the potential consequences. This can contribute to the development of resistant strains of bacteria, making it harder to find an effective treatment.

By being more mindful of antibiotic use and exploring natural alternatives, individuals can help combat antibiotic resistance and promote healthier outcomes for UTIs.

Natural remedies and lifestyle changes can be effective in treating UTIs without resorting to antibiotics. For example, increasing water intake can help flush out bacteria from the urinary tract, while consuming cranberry juice or supplements can prevent bacteria from adhering to the bladder walls. Additionally, incorporating probiotics into your diet can help maintain a healthy balance of bacteria in the gut and urinary tract, reducing the risk of infection.

It is important to consult with a healthcare provider before attempting to treat a UTI naturally, especially if you have a history of recurrent infections or underlying health conditions. They can help determine the best course of action for your specific situation and offer guidance on incorporating natural remedies into your treatment plan.

By taking a holistic approach to UTI management, you can reduce your reliance on antibiotics and help prevent the development of antibiotic resistance in the future.

In conclusion, antibiotic resistance is a serious issue that affects the treatment of UTIs. By being proactive about your health, exploring natural remedies, and working closely with healthcare providers, you can effectively manage UTIs without contributing to antibiotic resistance.

Remember to listen to your body, practice good hygiene, and prioritize your overall well-being to prevent UTIs and promote long-term healing.

Alternative therapies for UTI relief

If you are looking for alternative therapies to help relieve the symptoms of UTI, you have come to the right place. In this subchapter, we will discuss some natural remedies that can provide quick relief from the discomfort and pain associated with urinary tract infections. These alternative therapies are safe, effective, and can be used in conjunction with traditional medical treatments for UTI.

One alternative therapy for UTI relief is the use of probiotics. Probiotics are beneficial bacteria that can help restore the balance of good bacteria in your gut and urinary tract. By taking a probiotic supplement or eating probiotic-rich foods such as yogurt and kefir, you can help boost your immune system and fight off the harmful bacteria that cause UTIs.

Another natural remedy for UTI relief is drinking plenty of water. Staying hydrated is essential for flushing out bacteria from your urinary tract and preventing the infection from spreading. Aim to drink at least 8-10 glasses of water a day to help alleviate the symptoms of UTI and speed up the healing process.

Herbal remedies such as cranberry extract and D-mannose are also effective alternative therapies for UTI relief. Cranberry extract contains compounds that can prevent bacteria from sticking to the walls of the bladder, while D-mannose is a natural sugar that can help flush out bacteria from the urinary tract. These herbal remedies can be taken in supplement form or as a tea to help alleviate the symptoms of UTI.

In addition to probiotics, water, and herbal remedies, acupuncture and acupressure are alternative therapies that can help relieve the discomfort of UTI. Acupuncture involves inserting thin needles into specific points on the body to help restore the flow of energy and promote healing, while acupressure involves applying pressure to these same points to alleviate pain and inflammation. Both of these alternative therapies can be used in conjunction with traditional medical treatments for UTI to provide quick relief.

Overall, alternative therapies for UTI relief can be a safe and effective way to alleviate the symptoms of urinary tract infections. By incorporating probiotics, water, herbal remedies, acupuncture, and acupressure into your treatment plan, you can help speed up the healing process and prevent future UTIs from occurring. Always consult with a healthcare professional before starting any new alternative therapy to ensure it is safe and appropriate for your individual needs.

How To Heal UTI Naturally

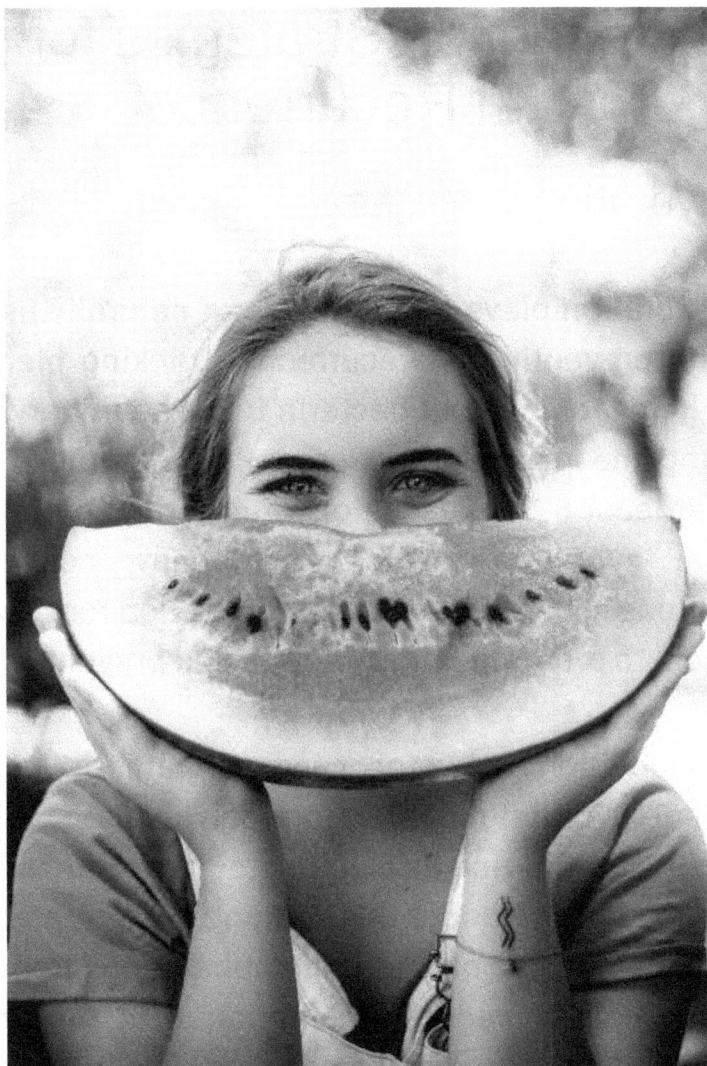

A Comprehensive Guide for Quick Recovery

Chapter 7

Prevention Strategies for UTI Recurrence

Hydration

Hydration plays a crucial role in naturally healing UTI and preventing its recurrence. Drinking plenty of water helps to flush out bacteria from the urinary tract, reducing the risk of infection. It is recommended to drink at least 8-10 glasses of water a day to maintain optimal hydration levels. Additionally, consuming herbal teas such as cranberry or dandelion root tea can also help to promote urinary health and prevent UTI.

In addition to water, coconut water is another excellent hydrating option for individuals with UTI. Coconut water is rich in electrolytes and antioxidants, which can help to boost the immune system and fight off infection. It also has natural antibacterial properties that can help to reduce inflammation in the urinary tract. Including coconut water in your daily hydration routine can be a refreshing and effective way to support your body's natural healing process.

Avoiding dehydrating beverages such as alcohol, caffeine, and sugary drinks is essential for individuals with UTI. These beverages can irritate the bladder and exacerbate symptoms of UTI. Instead, opt for hydrating options such as water, herbal teas, and coconut water to support your body's natural healing process. Maintaining proper hydration levels is key to preventing UTI and promoting overall urinary health.

Incorporating hydrating foods such as watermelon, cucumbers, and leafy greens into your diet can also support your body's hydration levels and promote urinary health. These foods have high water content and are rich in vitamins and minerals that can help to support the immune system and reduce inflammation in the urinary tract. Including a variety of hydrating foods in your diet can help to prevent UTI and support your body's natural healing process.

Overall, staying properly hydrated is essential for individuals with UTI. Drinking plenty of water, herbal teas, and coconut water, while avoiding dehydrating beverages, can help to flush out bacteria from the urinary tract and reduce the risk of infection.

Additionally, incorporating hydrating foods into your diet can support your body's hydration levels and promote urinary health. By prioritizing hydration, you can support your body's natural healing process and prevent UTI from recurring.

Proper hygiene

Proper hygiene is crucial when it comes to preventing and treating urinary tract infections (UTIs). UTIs are often caused by bacteria entering the urethra and multiplying in the bladder. By maintaining good hygiene practices, you can reduce your risk of developing a UTI and promote healing if you are currently experiencing one.

One of the most important aspects of proper hygiene for UTI prevention is staying clean and dry. This means wiping from front to back after using the bathroom to prevent bacteria from entering the urethra. It is also important to wear loose-fitting, breathable underwear and avoid wearing tight clothing that can trap moisture and create a breeding ground for bacteria. Keeping the genital area clean and dry can help prevent bacteria from multiplying and causing an infection.

In addition to staying clean and dry, it is important to drink plenty of water to help flush out bacteria from the urinary tract. Hydration is key in preventing UTIs and promoting healing if you already have one.

Drinking water can help dilute urine and make it less concentrated, reducing the likelihood of bacteria sticking to the bladder walls and causing an infection. Aim to drink at least eight glasses of water a day to maintain proper hydration and support urinary health.

Proper hygiene also extends to your choice of personal care products. Avoid using harsh soaps, perfumes, and douches in the genital area, as these can disrupt the natural balance of bacteria and increase your risk of developing a UTI. Opt for gentle, fragrance-free products that are specifically formulated for sensitive skin to help maintain a healthy environment in the urinary tract.

It is also important to change out of wet bathing suits and sweaty workout clothes promptly to prevent bacteria from thriving in moist environments.

In conclusion, proper hygiene is essential for preventing and healing UTIs naturally. By practicing good hygiene habits, such as staying clean and dry, drinking plenty of water, and using gentle personal care products, you can reduce your risk of developing a UTI and support your body's natural healing process if you are currently experiencing one.

Remember that prevention is key when it comes to UTIs, so make sure to prioritize your urinary health by incorporating proper hygiene practices into your daily routine.

Probiotic maintenance

Probiotic maintenance is an essential aspect of healing UTI naturally. Probiotics are live bacteria and yeasts that are good for your health, especially your digestive system. These friendly bacteria help maintain the balance of good and bad bacteria in your gut and urinary tract, which is crucial for preventing and managing UTIs.

One of the best ways to incorporate probiotics into your daily routine is by consuming probiotic-rich foods such as yogurt, kefir, sauerkraut, kimchi, and kombucha. These foods can help replenish the good bacteria in your gut and urinary tract, reducing the risk of UTIs and promoting overall gut health.

In addition to consuming probiotic-rich foods, you may also consider taking a high-quality probiotic supplement. Look for a supplement that contains a variety of probiotic strains, including Lactobacillus and Bifidobacterium, which are known for their beneficial effects on gut and urinary tract health.

It's important to note that not all probiotic supplements are created equal, so do your research and choose a reputable brand that has been tested for quality and efficacy.

Consult with your healthcare provider before starting any new supplement regimen, especially if you have any underlying health conditions or are taking medications.

By incorporating probiotic maintenance into your daily routine, you can help support your body's natural defenses against UTIs and promote overall urinary tract health. Remember that healing UTI naturally is a holistic process that involves taking care of your gut health, maintaining a healthy lifestyle, and working with your healthcare provider to find the best treatment plan for your individual needs.

Regular urination

Regular urination is an essential part of maintaining good urinary health, especially for those who suffer from UTIs. By emptying the bladder frequently, you can help flush out bacteria and prevent them from growing and causing infection. It is important to drink plenty of water throughout the day to ensure that you are able to urinate regularly. Aim for at least 8-10 glasses of water daily to stay hydrated and promote healthy urine flow.

If you are experiencing symptoms of a UTI, such as painful urination or a frequent urge to urinate, it is important to make sure you are emptying your bladder completely each time you go.

Holding in urine for extended periods of time can increase the risk of developing a UTI by allowing bacteria to multiply in the bladder. Make sure to take your time when urinating and relax to ensure that you are fully emptying your bladder.

In addition to regular urination, practicing good hygiene habits can also help prevent UTIs. Wiping from front to back after using the bathroom can help prevent bacteria from entering the urethra and causing infection.

It is also important to urinate before and after sexual activity to help flush out any bacteria that may have entered the urinary tract.

For those looking to heal a UTI naturally, regular urination is a key component of the treatment plan. By ensuring that you are emptying your bladder frequently, you can help reduce the concentration of bacteria in the urinary tract and promote healing. Remember to stay hydrated, practice good hygiene habits, and listen to your body's signals to ensure that you are urinating regularly and effectively.

In conclusion, regular urination is crucial for maintaining good urinary health and preventing UTIs. By emptying the bladder frequently, you can help flush out bacteria and prevent infection. Make sure to drink plenty of water, practice good hygiene habits, and listen to your body's signals to ensure that you are urinating regularly and effectively. By incorporating regular urination into your daily routine, you can help heal UTIs naturally and promote overall urinary health.

Stress management techniques

Stress management techniques play a crucial role in the overall healing process of UTI. Stress has been linked to weakening the immune system, making the body more susceptible to infections like UTI. By incorporating stress management into your daily routine, you can support your body's natural ability to fight off the infection and promote quicker relief.

One effective stress management technique is deep breathing exercises. By taking slow, deep breaths, you can activate the body's relaxation response, which can help reduce feelings of anxiety and stress. Practice deep breathing exercises for a few minutes each day to help calm your mind and body.

Another helpful stress management technique is mindfulness meditation. Mindfulness involves focusing on the present moment and accepting it without judgment.

By practicing mindfulness meditation, you can reduce stress, improve your mental clarity, and enhance your overall well-being. Take a few minutes each day to sit quietly and focus on your breath, bringing your attention back to the present moment whenever your mind starts to wander.

Engaging in physical activity is also a great way to manage stress and support the healing process of UTI. Exercise releases endorphins, which are natural mood-boosting chemicals that can help reduce stress and promote a sense of well-being.

Whether it's going for a walk, practicing yoga, or hitting the gym, find a physical activity that you enjoy and make it a regular part of your routine.

In addition to these techniques, maintaining a healthy diet, getting enough sleep, and staying hydrated are also important aspects of stress management and UTI healing. By taking a holistic approach to managing stress, you can support your body's natural ability to fight off infections and promote optimal healing. Remember to listen to your body, prioritize self-care, and seek support from healthcare professionals if needed.

How To Heal UTI Naturally

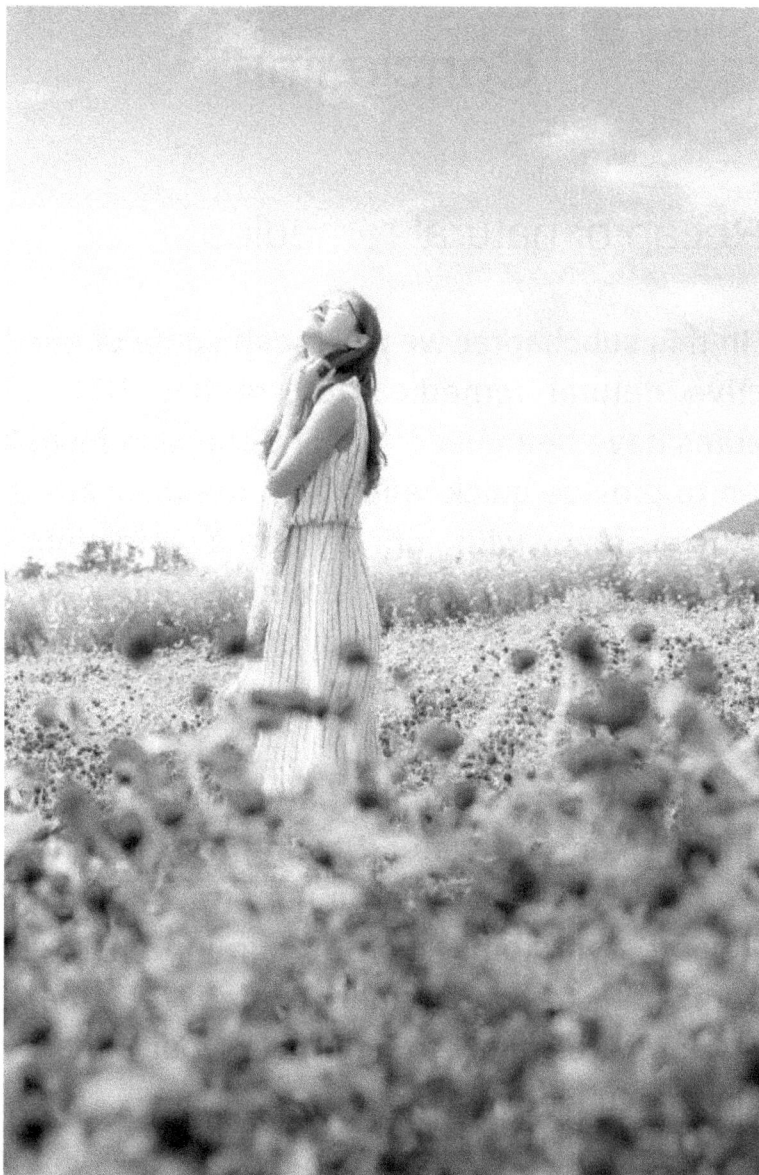

A Comprehensive Guide for Quick Recovery

Chapter 8

Conclusion

Recap of natural remedies

In this subchapter, we will recap some of the most effective natural remedies for treating UTI. These remedies have been used for centuries and have been proven to provide quick relief from the discomfort and pain associated with urinary tract infections. By incorporating these natural remedies into your daily routine, you can help your body fight off the infection and prevent it from recurring.

One of the most popular natural remedies for UTI is drinking plenty of water. Staying hydrated helps to flush out bacteria from your urinary tract and can help to alleviate symptoms such as burning and frequent urination. It is recommended to drink at least 8-10 glasses of water a day to help keep your urinary tract healthy and functioning properly.

Another effective natural remedy for UTI is cranberry juice. Cranberries contain compounds that can help to prevent bacteria from adhering to the walls of the urinary tract, making it easier for your body to flush them out. Drinking a glass of unsweetened cranberry juice daily can help to prevent and treat UTI.

Probiotics are also a great natural remedy for UTI. Probiotics are beneficial bacteria that help to maintain the balance of good bacteria in your gut and urinary tract. By taking a probiotic supplement or eating probiotic-rich foods such as yogurt and kefir, you can help to prevent UTI and promote overall urinary tract health.

Garlic is another natural remedy that has been used for centuries to treat infections, including UTI. Garlic contains compounds that have antibacterial and antifungal properties, making it an effective treatment for UTI. You can incorporate garlic into your diet by adding it to your meals or taking a garlic supplement to help fight off the infection.

Lastly, D-mannose is a natural remedy that can help to quickly relieve the symptoms of UTI. D-mannose is a type of sugar that can help to prevent bacteria from adhering to the walls of the urinary tract, making it easier for your body to flush them out. Taking a D-mannose supplement can help to alleviate symptoms such as burning and frequent urination and promote healing of the urinary tract.

By incorporating these natural remedies into your daily routine, you can help to heal UTI naturally and prevent it from recurring in the future.

Importance of lifestyle changes

In this subchapter, we will discuss the importance of lifestyle changes in healing UTI naturally. UTIs, or urinary tract infections, are common infections that can be both painful and uncomfortable. While antibiotics are often prescribed to treat UTIs, making lifestyle changes can help prevent future infections and promote overall urinary tract health.

One of the most important lifestyle changes you can make to heal UTI naturally is to stay hydrated. Drinking plenty of water helps flush out bacteria from the urinary tract and can help prevent infections from occurring. Aim to drink at least eight glasses of water a day, and avoid sugary drinks and caffeine, which can irritate the bladder and make UTI symptoms worse.

Another important lifestyle change to consider is maintaining good hygiene. This includes wiping from front to back after using the bathroom, wearing cotton underwear, and showering regularly. Poor hygiene can introduce bacteria into the urinary tract and increase the risk of developing a UTI. By practicing good hygiene habits, you can help prevent infections and promote urinary tract health.

Eating a healthy diet rich in fruits, vegetables, and whole grains can also help heal UTI naturally. Certain foods, such as cranberries, blueberries, and garlic, have been shown to have antibacterial properties and can help prevent UTIs. Avoiding processed foods, sugary snacks, and excessive alcohol consumption can also help reduce inflammation in the urinary tract and promote healing.

Lastly, managing stress and getting enough sleep are important lifestyle changes to consider when healing UTI naturally. Stress weakens the immune system and can make you more susceptible to infections, including UTIs.

Taking time to relax, practice mindfulness, and get plenty of rest can help boost your immune system and promote healing. By making these lifestyle changes, you can help prevent future UTIs and promote overall urinary tract health.

Continued self-care for UTI prevention

Continued self-care is essential for preventing UTIs from recurring. While the initial treatment may have provided relief, it is important to continue practicing good habits to keep your urinary tract healthy. One of the most important things you can do is to stay hydrated by drinking plenty of water throughout the day. This helps to flush out bacteria and prevent them from multiplying in your bladder.

In addition to staying hydrated, it is also important to maintain good hygiene practices. This includes wiping from front to back after using the bathroom to prevent bacteria from entering the urethra.

It is also important to urinate after sex to help flush out any bacteria that may have been introduced during intercourse. Avoiding products that can irritate the urinary tract, such as scented feminine hygiene products or douches, can also help prevent UTIs.

Eating a healthy diet rich in fruits, vegetables, and whole grains can also help prevent UTIs. These foods provide essential nutrients that support a healthy immune system, which is crucial for fighting off infections. Avoiding foods that are high in sugar and refined carbohydrates can also help prevent UTIs, as these foods can promote the growth of bacteria in the urinary tract.

In addition to diet and hydration, regular exercise can also help prevent UTIs. Exercise helps to improve circulation and boost the immune system, making it easier for your body to fight off infections.

It is also important to manage stress, as chronic stress can weaken the immune system and make you more susceptible to infections. Finding healthy ways to relax and unwind, such as meditation or yoga, can help reduce your risk of UTIs.

By practicing continued self-care and making healthy lifestyle choices, you can help prevent UTIs from recurring. Remember to stay hydrated, practice good hygiene, eat a healthy diet, exercise regularly, and manage stress. These simple habits can make a big difference in keeping your urinary tract healthy and preventing UTIs.

Resources for further information

If you are looking for more information on how to heal UTI naturally, there are several resources available to help guide you through the process. These resources can provide you with additional tips, advice, and support to help you find relief from your UTI symptoms.

One valuable resource for further information is the National Institute of Diabetes and Digestive and Kidney Diseases (NIDDK), which offers a wealth of information on UTIs, including causes, symptoms, and treatment options. Their website provides in-depth articles, fact sheets, and resources to help you better understand and manage your UTI.

Another helpful resource is the National Kidney Foundation, which offers a variety of resources for people suffering from UTIs and other kidney-related issues. Their website includes educational materials, support groups, and information on how to prevent UTIs in the future.

For those interested in natural remedies for UTIs, the book "Healing UTI Naturally: A Comprehensive Guide for Quick Relief" is an excellent resource. This book provides practical tips and advice on how to naturally heal UTIs, including dietary changes, lifestyle modifications, and herbal remedies.

Lastly, joining online forums and support groups for people with UTIs can be a great way to connect with others who are going through similar experiences. These communities can offer valuable insight, advice, and emotional support as you navigate your UTI healing journey. By utilizing these resources for further information, you can arm yourself with the knowledge and tools needed to effectively manage and heal your UTI naturally.

Final thoughts and encouragement

As you reach the end of this comprehensive guide on healing UTI naturally, I want to leave you with some final thoughts and words of encouragement. Dealing with a UTI can be incredibly frustrating and uncomfortable, but there are steps you can take to alleviate your symptoms and promote healing in a natural way.

First and foremost, it's important to remember that you are not alone in this journey. UTIs are a common condition that many people experience at some point in their lives.

By educating yourself on natural remedies and lifestyle changes that can help manage your symptoms, you are taking proactive steps towards improving your health and well-being.

It's also crucial to listen to your body and pay attention to any changes or new symptoms that may arise. UTIs can be stubborn infections that require patience and consistency in your treatment approach. If you are not seeing improvement or if your symptoms worsen, don't hesitate to seek medical advice from a healthcare professional.

Remember to stay hydrated and maintain good hygiene practices to prevent future UTIs. Drinking plenty of water and urinating frequently can help flush out bacteria and prevent infections from recurring. Additionally, incorporating probiotics, cranberry juice, and other natural remedies into your daily routine can help support your body's immune system and promote healing.

Lastly, I want to encourage you to approach your healing journey with a positive mindset and determination. It may take time to fully recover from a UTI, but by staying committed to your natural treatment plan and prioritizing self-care, you can find relief and restore your health. Trust in your body's ability to heal and know that you have the resources and support to overcome this challenge. Stay strong, stay positive, and remember that healing is possible.

Author Notes & Acknowledgments

First and foremost, I would like to express my deepest gratitude to the people who inspired and supported me throughout the journey of writing this book. This project would not have been possible without their unwavering belief in me and their invaluable contributions.

To my wife, thank you for your constant encouragement and understanding. Your love and support have been my anchor during the challenging times of researching and writing this book. Your belief in my ability to make a difference in people's lives has been my driving force.

I would also like to disclose that this book contains some renewed artificial intelligence-generated content. I really appreciate very recent technological innovation by outstanding scientists and of course our reader's understanding.

Lastly, I want to express my deepest gratitude to the readers of this book. I sincerely hope the strategies and methods outlined within these pages will provide you with the knowledge and tools needed to truly make your life much better. Your commitment to seeking any good solutions and willingness to explore multiple methods is commendable.

Author Bio

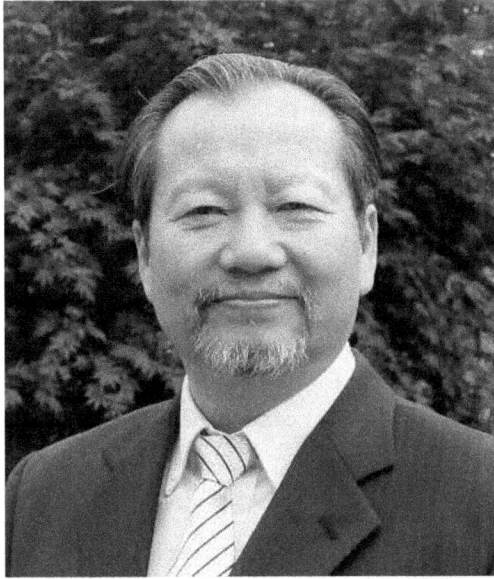

Johnson Wu earned his MD in 1982. With over 40 years of clinical experience, he has worked in hospitals in Zhejiang and Shanghai, China, as well as the Royal Marsden Hospital in London, UK.

Upon the recommendation of Sir Aaron Klug, the president of The Royal Society and a Nobel Prize winner in Chemistry, Dr. Wu was honorably awarded a British Royal Society Fellowship. He has published medical books and articles in seven countries and currently practices medicine in Canada.

Author Bio

www.ingramcontent.com/pod-product-compliance
Lightning Source LLC
Chambersburg PA
CBHW060251030426
42335CB00014B/1656